- https://exercise.trekeducation.org/assessment---rpe/
scale-rpe/
- https://themighty.com/2016/12/chronic-illness-uplifting-quotes/
- Guan WJ, Liang WH, Zhao Y, et al. Comorbidity and its impact on 1590 patients with COVID-19 in China: a nationwide analysis. Eur Respir J. 2020;55(5): 2000547.doi:10.13993003.00547-2020
- Herridge MS, Moss M, Hough CL, et al. Recovery and outcomes after the acute respiratory distress syndrome (ARDS) in patients and their family caregivers. *Intensive Care Med 2016; 42: 725-738*
- Elizabeth Moffett, *Conquering COPD*, 2020
- https://lunginstitute.com/blog/breath-fresh-air-walking-outdoors-lung-health/#:~:text=According%20to%20the %20National%20Heart,lungs%20will%20stay %20healthier%20longer.
- www.goldcopd.org
- www.headspace.com-meditation-anxiety
- https://www.eatingwell.com/recipe/267223/walnut-rosemary-crusted-salmon/
- https://www.allrecipes.com/cook/lindalmt/
- https://www.webmd.com/lung/copd/pulmonary-rehabilitation-for-copd
- https://www.nhlbi.nih.gov/health-topics/pulmonary-rehabilitation
- https://www.webmd.com/lung/covid-recovery-overview#1

INTRODUCTION

Have you or a loved one been told that you would benefit from Pulmonary Rehabilitation? If so, are you having a hard time locating or completing a Pulmonary Rehabilitation Program? If you answered yes to either of these questions, then this book is for you. I wrote this book to bridge the gap between needed healthcare and available healthcare resources. Post pandemic healthcare isn't what it used to be. For starters, there is more of a demand for Pulmonary Rehab, but less availability due to new challenges concerning rules and regulations. Top that off with public fear of contracting COVID-19 and you have a broken system. Whether you are recovering from COVID-19 or suffering from chronic illness such as Chronic Obstructive Pulmonary Disease (COPD), Emphysema, Asthma, Interstitial Lung Disease (ILD or IPF), or other breathing ailments, this program may just be the perfect fit for you! I've developed a comprehensive Home Pulmonary Rehabilitation Program that can be completed in the comfort of your own home! This is the first and only Interactive Pulmonary Rehabilitation Book on the market and my hope is that you get relief from it! Join me on this journey to better breathing!

"No matter how many times we burst into flames, we can always rise from the ashes." - Anonymous

Preface

The world as we know it will never be the same. The year 2020 brought with it an unimaginable pandemic. Most of us shudder at the mention of the name Coronavirus or COVID-19. Some of us have made it out of the other end of this pandemic unscathed while others, the majority; will be picking up the pieces for many years to come. This includes our healthcare workers and health-care system as a whole. COVID-19 illness and restrictions have made a huge, seemingly bottomless gap in our healthcare system and the available services that we can provide. The purpose of this book is to bridge the healthcare gap and provide much needed pulmonary rehabilitation to those recovering from COVID-19 or suffering from other breathing ailments like COPD, Emphysema, and Asthma. We went through it together and we will recover together! After all, it is in our nature as humans to rise like a phoe-nix from the ashes, stronger and more powerful than ever before! Join me on this journey to better breathing and better health. If you are reading from a printed copy of my book, then go to You-Tube and type "Breathe Better with Elizabeth" into the search en-gine. My page should come up. The video is titled "Welcome! We are on a journey to help you breathe better!" Click here to view my intro video: https://youtu.be/Un-hzXedpVE

> *"Hope is important because it can make the present mo-ment less difficult to bear. If we believe that tomorrow will be better, we can bear a hardship today." - Thich Nhat Hanh*

◆ ◆ ◆

Day 1 Orientation

It's orientation day!

SUPPLIES

- ❖ Journal

❖   1-3 lb weights (can substitute with soup cans or full water bottles if needed)
❖   Ankle weights
❖   Stress Ball
❖   Pulse-Oximeter
❖   Pedometer (not a necessity)

<u>EXERCISE</u>

Safety First! Before starting this program, it's imperative that you get approval from your Doctor. The benefit of participating in an in-person program is that you are supervised by medical professionals. For this program, in the absence of supervision, I'll be teaching you how to monitor yourself.

The key to exercising with breathing problems is not to overdo it. Most of us have been raised with the "What doesn't kill you makes you stronger mentality." This is not true when it comes to Pulmonary Rehabilitation! As you work out, I don't want it to feel too easy or too hard. I want you right in the middle. Here's an awesome chart to go by called the BORG Scale 1-10: https://exercise.trekeducation.org/assessment/borg-scale-rpe/ **I want you to stay between 3-5.** If you are at a 2, then increase what you're doing. If you're at a 6 or higher, then slow down and even stop if necessary. You will also need to check your blood oxygen level with your pulse-oximeter periodically. Especially if you're short of breath. Your blood oxygen level should be 92% or higher when you exercise. Don't exercise if your oxygen is less than 92% because you will not be doing yourself any favors. Your muscles need adequate oxygen to function properly and grow!

All of your exercises will be written with a corresponding video. ALL of the videos will be found on my personal YouTube Channel titled "Breathe Better with Elizabeth".

BORG SCALE 1-10 PERCEIVED EXERTION SCALE

0 - Rest
1 - Really Easy
2 - Easy
3 - Moderate
4 - Sort of Hard
5 - Hard
6 - Hard
7 - Really Hard
8 - Really Hard
9 - Really, Really, Hard
10 - Maximal:Just like my hardest race

Here are the signs/symptoms to watch for. Stop exercising if ANY of these occur:

- Breathlessness to the point that you cannot speak
- Chest pain, discomfort, or tightness
- Feeling dizzy or faint
- Leg pain or cramping

If these symptoms persist once you've rested, then please call your doctor.

JOURNALING

Journaling daily is such an important role in your journey that I urge you to commit to journaling daily for the next 21 days. Journaling will help you better understand your lungs as well as begin a healing process for your mind. So, I can hear you asking "How will journaling help me to better understand my lungs?" The answer is that everyone's lungs are different. What causes you to have increased shortness of breath may not be what causes the next person to become breathless. Everyone has unique "triggers" and once you've figured out what yours are, you can begin to avoid them! Now, to begin with, I want you to log your shortness of breath on a scale of 1-10 twice daily. When you're logging this I also want you to rate your mood on a scale of 1-10 as well. You will begin to notice a correlation between your mood and your breathing. This is very important when it comes to learning how to control your breathing. Watch for deviations or trends in your numbers. If your numbers become better or worse from one day to the next then you should stop and brainstorm. What have I eaten since my last entry? Where have I gone since my last entry? Was I exposed to anything different or new? I will also be giving you questions to reflect upon daily as well.

You may be a little bit overwhelmed right now and that's normal. This journey will not be an easy one, but it is a necessary one if you want to breathe better! Stay committed, stay strong, and become the warrior that I know you are. Let's do this!

Journal Day 1:

- ❑ Rate Breathing from 1-10
- ❑ Rate Mood from 1-10
- ❑ How do you feel about yourself?
- ❑ If you could change anything about yourself, what would it be?
- ❑ What do you hope to get out of this program?

☐ On a scale from 1-10, How committed are you to change?

PLUG IN

- Plug in to a support system
- Join a CLOSED Facebook Group by searching for a group where the members share the same illness. Request to join a group and they will welcome you with open arms. You can find the name of my group at the bottom! Here are the names of several others active and supporting groups:

- COVID-19 Recovery:
  - Breathe Better with COPD, Emphysema, and COVID-19 Recovery
  - Covid-19 Recovery and Support

- COPD and Emphysema Sufferers:
  - COPD / A WARM LOVING PLACE TO HANG OUT
  - COPD WARRIORS INFO, SUPPORT, LOVE LAUGHTER
  - COPD SUPPORT GROUP
  - HEALTHY LIVING WITH COPD (BETTERBREATHERS CLUB)
  - Breathe Better with COPD, Emphysema, and COVID-19 Recovery
  - LIFT UP - COPD SUPPORT GROUP

- ARDS Sufferers:
  - ARDS Support Page for Survivors and Families of Patients-Information Page

- Pulmonary Fibrosis (IPF)Sufferers:
  - Pulmonary Fibrosis Patient Support by Breathe Support
  - Pulmonary Fibrosis

*REQUEST TO JOIN OUR CLOSED FACEBOOK GROUP: BREATHE BETTER WITH COPD, EMPHYSEMA, AND COVID-19 RECOVERY. This is a private group with people who share the same goals as you! It's a great place to plug in! https://youtu.be/YVimfIcH1Bs

*Follow this Link to my YouTube Page "Breathe Better with Elizabeth" for lots of helpful videos:

https://www.youtube.com/c/BreatheBetterwithElizabeth

"Inhale Confidence, Exhale Doubt" - Unknown

Day 2 Back To The Breathing Basics

If you are reading this, then you have more than likely been battling with shortness of breath to some extent. Whether you are recovering from COVID-19 or battling a chronic illness, anyone with breathing problems can benefit from Pulmonary Rehabilitation. People come to Pulmonary Rehab with various lung problems and varying degrees of shortness of air, but the remedy is the same for everyone. I am going to teach you how to break the cycle of breathlessness, otherwise known as the Dyspnea Cycle.

You will break the cycle by retraining and strengthening your respiratory muscles as well as learning strategies that you will use in different situations. It will not be easy, but it will be worth it! The power to stop the cycle of breathlessness is within you.

Most people come to me when they are stuck in the Dyspnea Cycle. Dyspnea is a fancy word for a person's perceived shortness of breath. To put it simply, it's a vicious cycle that begins with you being short of breath - then your stress hormones like adrenaline kick in causing you to breathe more rapidly (making you anxious) - leading you to become more short of breath. This causes you to avoid certain situations or activities - which in turn cause you to become more sedentary (weakening your muscles). Then, when you go to do something, your muscles are weaker, requiring more oxygen to function - making you more short of air and anxious than when the cycle first started... and round and round it goes.

If your stress hormones kick in too often, your body's fight or flight mechanism (sympathetic nervous system) begins to stay on high alert, which causes anxiety and a slew of other problems including digestive issues. Unfortunately, anxiety also causes shortness of breath. As you can see, it is imperative that you learn to break this cycle!

Step one is to relearn how to breathe. Sounds simple, right? Not so fast. This takes discipline and lots of practice in order to regain control of your breath. You need to begin by consciously breathing in through your nose and out through your mouth. Breathing in through your nose actually has a couple of benefits. For starters, your nose acts as an air filter when you breathe in. It can trap certain particles on the way in that your mouth does not trap. On top of that, it is also a built in humidifier in that it moistens and warms the air as it comes in. In that one simple step, you are now filtering and humidifying your lungs!

The next step in relearning how to breathe is to slow your breathing down, especially when you are short of air. This is opposite of what your brain tells you to do. The problem with breathing faster as you get short of air is that you are not getting enough air into the parts of your lungs that the oxygen needs to get to. Slowing your breathing down is imperative to getting a nice, full, oxygen giving breath. If you are not used to breathing slowly, it will take lots and lots of practice to rewire your brain. In fact, you need to start practicing breathing exercises multiple times a day when you are not short of breath so it is easier for you to do when necessary.

Diaphragmatic breathing, otherwise known as belly breathing, is the first breathing exercise to master. The diaphragm is a muscle that sits directly underneath the lungs and above your stomach. It's the primary muscle that should be used when breathing. By the time people are referred to pulmonary rehabilitation, their diaphragm is usually weak and not being used. If you have COPD, Emphysema, or Asthma, your diaphragm may be flattened due to trapped air in your lungs pushing down on it. If you're recovering from COVID-19, have IPD, ILD, or ARDS then your diaphragm will be weak due to overuse. When your diaphragm is weak, your body begins to use other muscles (called accessory muscles) to breathe. The more muscles you use, the more energy and oxygen you use. Strengthening your diaphragm is crucial on your path to better breathing!

Diaphragmatic Breathing (Belly Breathing)

1. Sit comfortably with your feet touching the floor and back supported.
2. Place one hand on your chest and one hand on your stomach
3. Inhale (breathe in) through your nose while pushing your stomach out. You should feel the movement coming from your stomach rather than your chest.
4. Exhale (breathe out), pushing the air out of your lungs as you pull your stomach in

This probably will not feel natural at first and it may take a while to master, but do not get discouraged. You will get it, I promise! Some people find it beneficial to practice in front of a mirror until they get it down. You need to exercise your diaphragm 3-5 (or more) times a day. It is in fact a muscle and needs to be worked to build its strength. Once your diaphragm gets stronger, your breathing will begin to get a little easier. You may be tempted to stop practicing this method of breathing once you have mastered it, but please don't! You want to create muscle memory so that when you get short of breath, your mind and body naturally use this method of breathing.

If you have COPD or Emphysema, along with using your dia-phragm, you need to add "Pursed Lips" to your exhalation (breath-ing out). This is to prevent you from trapping air in your lungs, which can be a problem for people who suffer from either illness, as well as keeps your airways open longer for better gas (CO_2 & Oxygen) exchange. To do this, pucker your lips and breathe out slowly (twice as long as what you breathe in).

If you are recovering from COVID-19 or ARDS or you suffer from IPFor ILD, just breathe out normally through your mouth when you exhale.

To learn more about these methods and watch a demonstration do to my video titles "Breathe Better: Building Strength in your Dia-phragm" or click on the following link:
https://youtu.be/WHauAaI4wV0

Journal Day 2:

- □ Rate both Breathing and Mood separately on a scale from 1-10
- □ What steps do you need to take to correct your breathing?
- □ How will life be different for you if you can learn to control

your breathing?

"I cannot say whether things will get better if we change; what I can say is they must change if they are to get better."
- George C. Lichtenberg

◆ ◆ ◆

Day 3 The Power Of The Breath Part #1

Applying your new breathing techniques to your everyday life is essential in breaking the dyspnea cycle. There is power in the breath! I am going to teach you how to make your breath work for you rather than against you. The first technique is called Coordinated Breathing. This can be used anytime that you are performing a physically demanding task like lifting heavy objects or even walking up stairs. The key is to always take a nice deep breath in through your nose while you are at rest, then exhale during the difficult part of the task. There is power in the exhale! Take stares for example: Inhale through your nose as your feet are flat on the ground and then exhale through your mouth as you take a step up. Inhale through your nose when both feet are flat on the step and exhale through your mouth as you step up and so on and so. Now, let's say you're picking up a laundry basket full of clothes off of the floor. Inhale through your nose as you are standing straight up, then exhale through your mouth as you bend down AND pick up the basket. You will be amazed by how well these strategies work! I've included a video with demonstrations to help you to understand titles "". Click the link here: https://youtu.be/h2i5nSOTGDc Or go to my YouTube Page and Find the video Titled "Coordinated Breathing for COPD, Coronavirus..."

I also want you to add some gentle stretches to your daily breathing exercises. Gentle stretches will get your body ready for movement. Look up my video titled "Breathe Better: Gentle Daily Stretches for..." Click on the link here:
https://youtu.be/cAwkTO65-So

For those who prefer written instructions, I've included them as well.

Gentle Daily Stretches:

Neck Stretch
1. Begin seated in a straight-backed chair with your feet flat on the floor.
2. Pull your back away from the chair and sit up straight.
3. Breathe in slowly through your nose and exhale through your mouth as you gently bend your neck to the right (right ear facing down towards your shoulder)
4. Stays here for one breath and on an inhale bring your head back to center.
5. Repeat on the other side

Shoulder Roles

1. Gently roll your shoulders forward 5 times.
2. Gently roll your shoulders back 5 times.

Shoulder Drops

1. With your hand down by your side, gently drop your right shoulder (keeping your head and neck in line with your spine), moving your right hand towards the floor.
2. Hold for 1 full breath
3. Raise back up to sitting position
4. Repeat on your left side
5. Repeat both sides X 2

Seated Cat/Cow ***MY PERSONAL FAVORITE***

1. Gently arch your back, looking up to the ceiling as you breathe in through your nose.
2. Round your back as you exhale
3. Repeat X 4

Twists

1. Sit up straight and inhale through your nose
2. Slowly turn your upper body to the right, looking over your right shoulder as you exhale.
3. Inhale as you come back to the starting position.
4. Slowly turn your upper body to the left, looking over your left shoulder as you exhale.
5. Inhale as you come back to the starting position
6. Repeat X 2 on each side.

Journal Day 3:

- ❑ Rate both Breathing and Mood from 1-10
- ❑ Is the Diaphragmatic (Belly) Breathing getting any easier for you?
- ❑ Are you happy?

- ❑ Make a list of things that make you happy.
- ❑ Make a list of things that you're thankful for.

"Breath is the link between mind and body." - *Dan Brule*

◆ ◆ ◆

Day 4 The Power Of The Breath Part #2

Coordinated breathing is great to use to prevent you from getting short of air (or more short of air during a task), but what about when you ARE short of air. Remember that the more muscles that you use, the more energy and oxygen you use. Therefore, when you get short of breath the very first thing you do is sit down or lean against a wall, taking pressure off as many of your muscles as possible. That way you do not use any more oxygen than necessary. This sounds like a no brainer, but the tendency of most people is to attempt to hurry and finish whatever it was that they were doing and THEN sit down. I can't stress this enough, stopping the shortness of breath before it's gone too far is crucial to your recovery! Breathing is far more important than anything else that you have going on. On top of sitting down, you should also relax your muscles as much as possible while you begin to focus on your breathing. Now you want to start the slow, deep breathing; in through your nose and out your mouth. Stay in this position until you have regained control of your breathing. Here is the link to my demonstration: https://youtu.be/D7IkqA0CHrI Or look up my video titled "Fast Facts with Elizabeth: What do I do when I get shortness of breath?"

<u>Step-by-Step:</u>

1. Stop what you are doing and sit down
2. If you happen to be in a store when this occurs, grab a shopping cart and lean on it to take pressure off your legs

3. If you don't have a cart, lean against a wall
4. Once you've settled in a comfortable position, relax your muscles (the best you can) and try to relieve any tension that you feel in your neck and shoulders
5. Begin deep breathing, in through your nose and out through your mouth, while slowing your breathing
6. Stay here until you've regained control of your breath

Journal Day 4:

- ❑ Rate both your Mood and Breathing from 1-10.
- ❑ Have you been active in any of your FB groups?
- ❑ If so, have you learned any good pointers for managing your breathing?

"Believe in yourself and all that you are. Know that there is something inside of you that is greater than any obstacle." - Christian D. Larson

Day 5 Hard Core Breathing Exercises

By now, you know the proper way to breathe and how to put it into practice. Today I am going to go over breathing exercises that will help you build strength in your diaphragm as well as the remaining core of your body. It is essential that you have a strong core for stability and good posture. It's much easier for your entire body to function, if your core is strong. You will breathe easier with a strong core. The exercises that we will go over today need to be practiced **every other day**. Like the diaphragmatic breathing exercise you have already learned, these exercises need to be continued even after you are breathing better to maintain strong muscles. Below, you will find written instruction, but if you prefer to do them with me you can look up the video titled "Breathe Better: Hard Core Breathing Exercises" or simply click on this link: https://youtu.be/VDAK4KaH2Gw

<u>Open & Close</u>
1. Sit in a comfortable position with your feet flat on the floor
2. Reach your arms straight out in front of you, palms touching
3. Inhale through your nose as your arms open wide into a T position
4. Exhale as your arms come back together
5. Without dropping your arms, repeat X 4

<u>Butterfly</u>
1. Sit in a comfortable position with your feet flat on the floor
2. Place your hands behind your head, elbows pointing out, even with your shoulders
3. Inhale through your nose, pushing your belly out
4. Exhale slowly as you bend forward, head towards your knees, elbows in towards your face
5. Inhale through your nose as you bring your body back to an upright position
6. Repeat X 4

<u>Active Twist</u>
1. Sit in a comfortable position with your feet flat on the floor
2. Reach your arms out straight by your sides into a T position
3. Inhale through your nose, pushing your stomach out
4. Exhale as your body twists to the right while your body remains in a T position

5. Inhale as you come back to center
6. Exhale as your body twists to the left while your body remains in a T position
7. Inhale back to center
8. Repeat X 4 on each side

Side Bend

1. Sit in a comfortable position with your feet flat on the floor
2. Place your hands behind your head, elbows pointing out, even with your shoulders
3. Inhale through your nose, pushing your belly out
4. Exhale slowly as you bend your torso to the right, right elbow facing the floor to the right
5. Inhale as you rise back up to initial position
6. Exhale slowly as you bend your torso the left, left elbow facing the floor to the left
7. Inhale as you rise back up
8. Repeat X 4 on each side

Knee to Chest

1. *This exercise is only for people who do not have difficulty lying flat their backs.*
2. Lie flat on your back (may add a pillow behind your head if needed) with both legs bent, feet flat on the bed
3. Inhale through your nose, pushing your belly out
4. Exhale slowly as you activate your abdominal muscles and bring your right knee to your chest (may use your hands for support if needed)
5. Inhale through your nose as you slowly lower your right leg
6. Exhale slowly, activating your abdominal muscles and bring your left knee to your chest (may use your hands for support if needed)
7. Inhale through your nose as you lower your left leg to the bed

8. Repeat X 4

<u>Journal Day 5</u>:

- ❏ Rate both Breathing and Mood from 1-10
- ❏ How is your diaphragmatic breathing now com   pared to when you first started only 4 short days ago?
- ❏ On a personal note, what are some needs of yours that aren't being met?
- ❏ Will breathing better help you meet any of those needs?
- ❏ If not, could you reach out to a family member or friend for help?

"I fight for my health every day in ways that most people don't understand. I am not lazy, I am a warrior!" - Unknown

Day 6 The Energy Exchange

When you suffer from a long term or chronic breathing illness, you must look at energy different from people who do not. Your bodies work harder all day, every day to keep up with the demands of your daily lives. Your body is using more energy than others are with every single breath. You probably cannot function the way you did in your younger years when breathing was not a daily battle for you. That being said, you should not have to stop doing anything that you love or enjoy just because your lungs are not as good as they used to be. Let us revisit the concept of working smarter, not harder. It is best to conserve your energy whenever possible so that you have it in times or situations that you know you will need it. I want you to continue doing the things that you love, but you may need to execute them differently. For example, if you love to shop, try to find stores with the motorized carts or at the very least always use a shopping cart to lean on for support. Bring your rescue inhaler or rescue nebulizer with you and take it 15 minutes before you plan to shop so that the medicine is in your system. I hear from people all of the time that they are too embarrassed to wear their oxygen out in public or use a motorized cart while shopping. Please do not let pride override your right to live a normal life!

Helpful hints for conserving your energy:

- Planning is EVERYTHING! At the beginning of every week, grab a calendar and a notebook so that you can tentatively plan your week. In your notebook, make 2 columns with the following titles: Have To, and Want to. Now, fill your columns with the activities for the upcoming week. Try to accomplish at least one necessity a day, spreading them out throughout the week. If you are having an awesome breathing day, then check out your list and complete a Want!
- Always allow yourself enough time. When you hurry and rush around it is much easier to hold your breath and forget to breathe. In addition, rushing increases your anxiety, which will make it harder to breathe.
- Recruit help; there is nothing wrong with asking for help. Can someone run errands for you, prepare a meal, or help you

clean up? After all, everyone needs a little help from time to time. I am confident that people will want to help you if you express your needs to them!

- Work slowly, focusing your breathing as you complete a task. Hurrying will cause more shortness of breath every time!
- Rest whenever you feel the need to, taking frequent breaks
- Avoid bending over. Try to keep the most frequently used items level with you rather than on the floor. Use a Grabbing Tool whenever you can. Bending over uses a ton of energy that you simply do not need to use.
- Avoid reaching up. Again, another reason to keep the majority of your belongings at a comfortable reach. Reaching up over your head also requires a ton of energy that you could otherwise save.
- Pull up a chair! Sit down for any activity that you can sit for. For example, bring your laundry to the bed or couch rather than hanging it up and folding it straight from the dryer. Pull up a stool when washing dishes or even cooking!
- If shopping is a problem for you, then always use a motorized cart if there is one available.
- Wear clothes with buttons in the front so that you are not reaching above your head to dress and undress.
- Try using a robe after a shower rather than drying off your body with a towel.

The exercises today will focus on balance and coordination. If you struggle with of these, then add either this video to your daily or every other day routine. For safety purposes, do them in the corner of a room or next to something that you can hold on to for stability. You can practice them with me on YouTube with video titled "Breathe Better Coordination and Balance Exercises" or clicking on the following link: https://youtu.be/X9C6FoX8wao

STRESS BALL
1. Begin squeezing your stress ball daily to improve grip strength and coordination. You can add this simple

exercise throughout your day as much or as little as needed.

2. Try sticking it in a place that you frequent like the kitchen table or your favorite chair!

THUMB TOUCH

1. While looking down at your right hand begin touching your thumb to your fingers one finger at a time.
2. Do this forward and backward before switching hands.
3. Repeat on your left hand.
4. Repeat both sides X 2
5. If this is super easy, then try doing it without looking at your hand!

STANDING

1. Stand with both feet flat on the floor about shoulder width apart.
2. Without holding on to anything, stand in one spot for 30-45 seconds.
3. If this is easy for you, then skip to the next exercise

TIGHTROPE WALK

1. Without holding on to anything, begin walking slowly, heal-to-toe.
2. You can place your arms out into a T position if it helps you to balance.
3. Walk as straight as possible for the length of a long hall.
4. Repeat each direction several times if possible

FOOT RAISE

1. Holding on to the wall or a chair, gently lift your right leg off of the floor.
2. Attempt to release your hold on the wall or chair for 5 seconds
3. Lower your right foot to the ground.
4. Holding on the wall or a chair, gently lift your left leg off of the floor

5. Attempt to release your hold on the wall or chair for 5 seconds.
6. Lower your left foot to the ground
7. Repeat on each side X 2

SIDE STEP

1. Facing a wall or counter top, step to the right with your feet shoulder width apart.
2. Bring your left foot to touch your right.
3. Continue walking sideways the length of the wall to the right
4. Repeat to the left side

Journal Day 6:

❑ Rate both Breathing and Mood from 1-10
❑ What activities have you stopped doing since your breathing problems began?
❑ Can you alter them so that you could do them again?
❑ Begin making a plan to do something that you would like to do again! The key is in the planning!

"I believe and therefore anything is possible." - *Unknown*

Day 7 Rest, Relaxation, And Reflection

Congratulations on completing your first week! I have thrown many concepts, education, and tasks at you and you are still here! The beauty of this program is that you do not have to actually follow the days to a Tee. This program is all about progress rather than perfection! If it takes you 2 days to get through Day 3, do not beat yourself up. You will have good days and bad days just like everyone else. The key is to finish the program, even if it takes you longer than the allotted 21 days. That being said, the people who put in the daily work see the best results. You need to be doing your breathing exercises every day! Let us recap what you have accomplished this week.

- You have plugged into a supportive Facebook Group.
- You have learned strategies to stop the cycle of shortness of breath.
- You have learned breathing exercises & techniques.
- You are strengthening your breathing muscles (Daily).
- You are improving your balance and coordination by doing exercises (Every other day).
- You have learned how to conserve energy.

Journal Day 7:

- Rate your Mood and Breathing from 1-10
- What has been your favorite day of the week and why?

- What is the most helpful thing you have learned this week?
- What is the driving force behind you completing this program?

"Always remember to fall asleep with a dream and wake up with a purpose." - Unknown

◆ ◆ ◆

Day 8 The Power Of Your Body

Exercise capacity gets worse with each day of inactivity. Your body adapts and does what you teach it to do. It is **within your power** to have a healthy body. Beginning an exercise routine is one of the most important things that you can do to battle shortness of breath. Your body functions better as a whole when you exercise. The stronger that your muscles are, the more efficient they are at using oxygen. Simply put, strong muscles utilize less oxygen than weak muscles. That is why the stronger your muscles are, the easier it is for you to complete tasks. Even walking is much easier and uses less oxygen when your core and legs are strong! Exercise releases endorphins, which help combat anxiety and depression. It helps to relieve muscle tension, improves circulation, and improves your sleep. Along with all of that, it will help you lose weight, decrease your blood pressure, help stabilize blood sugars, and lower your heart rate. On top of everything else, you will have increased energy to do things and you will feel better doing them!

I know what you are thinking, "Sure this sounds good in theory, but I have a hard time walking from the living room to the kitchen. How does she expect me to exercise?" I am going to tell you. You start small and build up weekly. We will start with seated exercises, and then add weights to the seated exercises, and then we will begin standing exercises and begin a walking program. Exercise comes in many different forms and I strongly encourage you to try them all! It can actually be really fun! Walking is probably the best exercise all around. It is easier on your joints, you can control the pace, you do not need any expensive equipment or gym membership, and it can be done using a cane or walker if needed.

Rules to Follow when Exercising:

- Have a bottle or glass of water nearby.
- Stretch both before and after a workout.
- Make sure that you can see the BORG Scale. I recommend making a small one of your own to keep out when needed.
- Keep a pulse-oximeter handy for when you get short of breath so you can check your oxygen level.
- Wait an hour after eating before exercising.
- Begin the exercises with no weights for the first time. If the movements are easy for you, then add 1 lb weights and build up until you reach 3 lbs. If you do not have access to hand weights, substitute soup cans or bottles of water.
- Stop exercising and rest if you reach 6 on the BORG Scale.
- Complete strengthening exercises 3 days a week.

Look up "Breathe Better Gentle Seated Exercises..." or follow this link to Gentle Home Exercises https://youtu.be/0WQwIqpSnsk

Begin by sitting up in a straight-backed chair with your feet flat on the ground and hands resting on your thighs.

SIDE STRETCH

1. Raise your right hand into the sky while holding on to your chair with your left hand.
2. Inhale through your nose and exhale as you reach your right hand over your head towards the opposite wall until you feel a stretch in your side.
3. Inhale as you come back up and release your arm.
4. Repeat this on your left side.
5. Do this on each side X 3

SHOULDER ROLLS

1. Roll shoulders in one direction for 10, switch

SHOULDER SHRUGS

1. Lift your shoulders up and down X 5

GENTLE NECK STRETCH

1. Sitting up straight, slowly tilt your head to the right, bringing your right ear to your right shoulder until you feel a stretch in the left side of your neck.
2. Hold for 5 seconds.
3. Repeat on the other side.
4. Do both sides X 3

SIDE BEND

1. Sit in a comfortable position with your feet flat on the floor
2. Place your hands behind your head, elbows pointing out, even with your shoulders
3. Inhale through your nose, pushing your belly out
4. Exhale slowly as you bend your torso to the right, right elbow facing the floor to the right
5. Inhale as you rise back up to initial position

ARM CIRCLES

1. Bring your arms out to a T shape.
2. Move your arms in a circular motion. The circles should be small, like the size of a dinner plate.
3. Do 10 in circles in each direction
4. Repeat X 3, resting in between if needed

ABDUCTIONS

1. Using a 1 lb weight, Bring arms out to a T shape and gently release back down.
2. Do this X 10

BICEP CURLS

1. With or without light weights, drop your arms to your side with palms facing forward
2. Gently curl your arms up by keeping your elbows close to your sides and bending your elbows
3. Do these X 20

SEATED ROWING

1. Sit up straight with your feet firmly on the floor.
2. Reach your arms out in front of you and clasp your hands together with your arms straight.
3. Pull your arms back to one side in a rowing motion with abdominal muscles engaged
4. Repeat on the other side.
5. Do X 10 on each side

KNEES UP

1. Sit up straight with your feet firmly on the floor.
2. Hold on to the sides of your chair with your hands.
3. Inhale through your nose while feet are flat on the floor.
4. As you begin to exhale, slowly lift your right foot off of the floor, towards your chest
5. Inhale through your nose as you gently place your right foot back on the floor
6. Exhale as you lift your left foot off the floor, toward your chest
7. Inhale through your nose as you drop your feet back to the floor.
8. Do each side X 10 (add ankle weights if this movement is too easy)

SEATED KICKS

1. Kick one leg out keeping it straight
2. Hold it out for 5 seconds.
3. Repeat on the other side
4. Do each side X 10 (add ankle weights if this is movement is too easy)

CALF RAISES

1. Sit up straight with the balls of your feet on the floor.
2. Left your heels from the ground while keeping your toes on the floor.
3. Hold for 5 seconds and lower them back down
4. Do this X 20

TOE RAISES

1. Lift your toes to the sky while leaving your heels on the floor.
2. Hold for 5 seconds and lower them back down.
3. Do this X 20

CALF STRETCH

1. Remaining seated, slide your right foot away from you until your right leg is straight and your right heel is resting on the floor.
2. Pull the toes on your right foot back towards your shins
3. Lean slightly forward from the hips
4. Repeat on the other side
5. Repeat X 2 on each side

HIP ABDUCTION

1. Sit up straight with both feet on the floor.
2. Move your legs wide apart and then together again.
3. Repeat X 10

SIDE STRETCH

1. Hold on to your chair with your left hand.
2. Raise your right arm towards the ceiling and reach for the opposite wall as you lean slightly to the left.
3. Hold for 5 seconds.
4. Drop your right arm and place it on the chair.
5. Raise your left arm towards the ceiling and reach for the opposite wall as you lean slightly to the right.
6. Hold for 5 seconds.
7. Drop your left arm.
8. Repeat X 2 on each side.

WAIST TWIST
1. Sit up straight with both feet flat on the floor.
2. Inhale through your nose pushing your stomach out.
3. Slowly exhale as you turn your upper body to the right, looking over your right shoulder.
4. Inhale as you return to the center.
5. Slowly exhale as you turn your upper body to the left, looking over your left shoulder.
6. Inhale as you return to the center.
7. Repeat X 2 on each side.

Journal Day 8 :

- ❑ Rate your Mood and Breathing from 1-10.
- ❑ How do you feel after exercising?
- ❑ Was it easy? Hard?
- ❑ How many days a week can you commit to exercising?

"The best way to get started is to quit talking and begin doing." - Walt Disney

Day 9: Maximizing Medications

Medicine is everywhere. If you go to the doctor for any ailment, you will more than likely leave with a prescription of some sort. On top of that, they may have also thrown some samples your way for the latest and greatest new medicine on the market! The problem with most samples is that they work really well, but cost a small fortune when it is time to pay for them monthly. This puts the majority of the population at a financial disadvantage. The biggest problem with this is that there are people who stop taking their breathing medications because they are too expensive. I want to teach you how to get the biggest bang for your buck! What doctors or pharmacists neglect to mention is that the older medications are cheaper and still effective! For instance, the nebulizer equivalent to any inhaler is cheaper than the inhaler version. It is less convenient, but more affordable and just as effective! In the appendix, you will find a conversion chart of new inhalers and their equivalents in nebulizer forms in case money is an issue.

While I do not believe that medication should be the only treatment for your ailments, I do believe that for people who have difficulty breathing, medication is a necessity for you to have a good quality of life. After all, it's no fun being short of breath. The first step is to know exactly what breathing medications that you are on and know what category of breathing meds that they fall under. It is important to note that a majority of your inhalers have more than one medication in it.

There are 3 main types of breathing medications:
- ❖ Bronchodilators (Both short and long acting), short acting are considered "Rescue Medications" to use when you're having a very hard time breathing, while the long acting are considered "Maintenance Medications" are you used to keep your airways open at all times
- ❖ Inhaled steroids; these work on the underlying inflammation of your lungs. These are very important! It takes several weeks of taking them regularly for them to begin working. A Lot of people make the mistake of thinking that they're not working because they can't feel them working like they can the bronchodilators, but please don't stop taking them!
- ❖ Combination (typically an inhaled steroid mixed with a long acting bronchodilator)

While these 3 groups can also be broken down into subcategories, for the purpose of simplicity, we'll stick with these 3. All of the medications are available in 1 of 3 forms; metered dose inhaler (MDI), dry powder inhaler (DPI), or nebulizer (NEB). While all 3 are equally effective, the nebulizer form works better for some because it's easier to take correctly. Most people are given these medications with little to no explanation on the proper technique to use them. If they are not taken correctly, then you are likely not getting all of the medication in the lungs, but rather in the back of your throat or tongue. Below you will find the proper way to take your medication. I have included an instructional video from another one of my books titled "How to take Breathing Medicine":

https://youtu.be/VheqfkL7AAO

TIPS
- Always take your maintenance medications at the same time every day. If the directions say Daily, then take it every 24 hours. If they say twice daily, take every 12 hours. This will allow the medication to stay in your system at all times.
- Try to avoid taking your rescue medications with your maintenance medications. Try to spread them out at least 3 hours before or after.
- Always use an aero chamber (spacer) with your inhalers! You will always get more medication when using one. If you do not have one, call your doctor and have them send an order for one to your pharmacy.
- Always rinse your mouth out after taking an inhaled steroid.

NEBULIZER: The nebulizer may be less convenient and take the longest, but I have always felt like they work better for patients because of their ease of use compared to an inhaler.
1. Place the medicine inside the nebulizer. Try to avoid contaminating the area that holds the medication.
2. Once turned on the nebulizer will begin to mist.
3. Place the mouthpiece in your mouth and begin to breathe in slowly through your mouth.
4. Exhale through the mouthpiece.
5. Every 3rd breath, take a deep breath in and hold it for 10 seconds before slowly letting it back out.
6. Repeat this until the nebulizer stops misting.

MDI (METERED DOSE INHALER)
1. Not all inhalers are the same, so it is important to read your directions that come with your specific inhaler.
2. Your MDI is under pressure and should not be kept or used near an open flame.

3. MDI's should ALWAYS be used with a Spacer or Holding Chamber. Using this prevents medication from escaping out of your mouth or into the air. It also prevents the medication from hitting the back of your throat. If you don't own a spacer, ask your Dr. for a prescription for one and you can pick it up from the pharmacy. *If you do not have any way of acquiring a spacer, you can use the tubing from the inside of a roll of toilet paper. I would only recommend this use short term until you can get your hands on the real thing."

4. Take the cap off your MDI, and then shake the canister well before each puff.

5. Place the mouthpiece of the inhaler into the spacer or tubing.

6. Sit or Stand up straight and completely empty your lungs by exhaling all of your air out.

7. Place the spacer in your mouth and make sure that your tongue does not block the flow of medicine.

8. Press down on the MDI and slowly inhale, filling your lungs from the bottom to the top.

9. Once your lungs are full, hold your breath for 10 seconds.

10. Take the spacer out of your mouth and exhale into the air.

11. Wait 60 seconds before taking the second puff (assuming your prescription calls to take a second puff).

12. Repeat steps 3-10.

13. When you are finished, rinse your mouth and spit.

14. Follow the directions on the package to clean and store the inhaler and spacer.

DPI (Dry Powdered Inhaler)

1. These come in different shapes and sizes, but mostly in a diskus

2. Hold it in one hand and put the thumb of your other hand on the thumb grip.

3. Push the thumb grip away until you hear a click. (Some DPIs require you to twist them until you hear a click). The sound of the click tells you that your dose is loaded.

4. Breathe completely (not into the DPI as this moisture can damage the med or device).

5. Inhale quickly and fully through the mouthpiece while sit-

ting up tall.
6. Hold your breath for 10 seconds, and then exhale into the air.
7. Rinse your mouth out.

INHALER TIPS
1. Always keep these in a cool, dry place away from direct sunlight.
2. Use them in an upright position.
3. Never skip a dose, even if you feel great. These medicines take time to build up in your system and need to stay in your system for maximum benefit. It is a common mistake for people to stop taking their inhalers when they feel better.
4. Never take an extra dose unless your doctor tells you to use it as needed.

Journal Day 9:
❑ Rate your Mood and Breathing from 1-10.
❑ Write your breathing medications down and write what category they fall under.
❑ What changes can you make to maximize your medications?

"Life is not about waiting for the storm to pass but learning to dance in the rain." - Unknown

◆ ◆ ◆

Day 10 Seeking, Finding, And Avoiding Triggers

Triggers are factors from your environment that can prompt an onset of symptoms related to breathing difficulty. If you have had breathing problems for a long time, then you may already know what your triggers are. Triggers are different from one person to the next so they can be hard to pinpoint. It is imperative that you do so though. If you know what your triggers are, then you can limit, or possibly even avoid them altogether. To do that, you must identify them.

Identifying your triggers is where that journal will come in handy. Remember that you are now tracking your breathing daily. Have you noticed any major changes from one day to the next? If so, it is possible that you were exposed to one of your triggers in that time period. Continue to keep track of your breathing score. If you notice a change in your breathing, then think back to where you have been and what you have eaten. You should also check allergen indexes. Over time, you will begin to notice patterns and from the patterns, you can identify your triggers. In general, any seasonal allergy that causes you to create more mucus can be a trigger for your lungs as well.

Common triggers
- Smoke from a cigarette or pipe
- Second hand smoke
- Smoke from a wood burning fireplace
- Third hand smoke

- Any other air pollution
- Anxiety
- Stress
- Season change
- Weed pollen
- Ragweed
- Mold
- Grass
- Perfumes
- Cleaning products, especially containing bleach
- Pet dander
- Cockroaches
- Dust
- Dust mites
- Dirty carpet, curtains, rugs, or upholstery
- Cold weather

Hints to control triggers

- Stay away from ALL forms of smoke
- Stay inside with the windows closed whenever possible
- Keep your house free from cockroaches and dust
- If you have pets, vacuum often and don't let them in the room where you sleep
- Wash sheets and pillows often in hot water
- Take allergy medications if prescribed by your doctor
- Use bleach free cleaning products
- Wear a scarf around your mouth in the cold

Journal Day 10:

- ❑ Rate your Mood and Breathing from 1-10.
- ❑ What are your possible triggers?
- ❑ What are some changes that you can make to avoid your triggers?
- ❑ Do you feel like you're mastering your breathing exercise yet?

"The secret of health for both mind and body is not to mourn for the past, not to worry about the future, or not to anticipate troubles, but to live the present moment wisely and earnestly." - Buddha

◆ ◆ ◆

Day 11 Coping With A Difficult Diagnosis

Whether you are recovering from COVID19 or dealing with another chronic illness like COPD. Coming to terms with a difficult diagnosis can be... well, difficult. It is completely normal to think, "Why me". You may be scared, sad, confused, or all of the above. Everyone copes differently so there is no right or wrong way to handle a difficult diagnosis. Any way that you look at it, it is downright frightening to lose the ability to breath. This can cause both depression and anxiety. That is why it is essential to your health that you learn to cope with your new reality. As I have already discussed, anxiety will only make matters worse. So, what is the solution?

For starters, you need to educate yourself on your condition. You can find anything and everything on the internet, which is not always a good thing. If you plan to research your condition on the internet, I urge you to stick with reputable websites like; Web MD or The Cleveland Clinic. On top of that, make a list of questions to take with you to your doctor. If they are not written down, then you may forget some of them. You should also write down your doctors responses as well. Being educated is empowering!

Another way to cope is through developing a support system. Your support system can be family, friends, or strangers from an online support group. They will all have different perfectives, which will all be useful in different ways. Your family and friends may not know what you are going through so it is your job to tell them. That is what they are there for. Your online support group is a perfect way to learn from others who have experienced similar things, share ideas, and find encouragement! You can develop lifelong friendships in support groups and may even be able to help others along the way. Helping others is a great way to heal If your needs are greater than what these avenues can provide, then please seek help from a mental health professional because no one should go through difficult times on their own.

More helpful tips:
- Stay active (which you are well on your way to doing)
- Daily meditation (may already be doing)
- Get up and get dressed every day
- Stay involved in hobbies or activities
- Get a good night sleep
- Maintain your relationships with family and friends (answer phone calls, return emails, and reciprocate invitations)
- Be a good listener (real relationships are a two way street)

Journal Day 11:

- Rate your Mood and Breathing from 1-10
- How do you feel you are coping with your diagnosis?
- What steps can you take to improve your ability to cope?
- How can you help someone else this week?
- Reach out to someone who has helped you along the way and let him or her know your appreciation.

"Your mind is a powerful thing. When you fill it with positive thoughts, your life will start to change." - *Unknown*

Day 12 Depression And Post Intensive Care Syndrome

Depression is seen in one form of the other with most people who have recovered from COVID-19 or are currently dealing with a chronic breathing problem This is especially true for people who have had lengthy hospital stays. This is due to several factors including, but not limited to; long-term hospital stays, isolation, loss, financial hardships, and fear of what the future holds. We will be going over some of them today, but know that if you have any of these symptoms, then it is imperative to seek help from a mental health professional. I cannot stress this enough. You must be your own health advocate in this day and time because no one else will do it for you! The medical community is overwhelmed with people needing help so it is common for healthcare team members to inadvertently overlook symptoms at an office follow up appointment. Please be sure to reach out if needed.

Common signs of symptoms of depression:
- Feeling of sadness
- Fatigue
- Sleep disturbances
- Trouble concentrating
- Feeling bad about yourself
- Hopelessness
- Poor appetite
- Overeating

- Thoughts of suicide

Have you had to be hospitalized during your treatment? If so, then you are even more at risk for depression. For starters, hospitals have been mandating limited to no visitors, which further isolates those who are ill. Being hospitalized by yourself can become very lonely, very quickly. Not only are your family and friends banned from visiting, but hospital staff have been advised to limit their contact with you as well. That would make even the brightest of minds turn dark.

If you or your loved one spent any length of time in the Intensive Care Unit (ICU), then it is possible that you could be suffering from Post-Intensive Care Syndrome. Post-Intensive Care Syndrome is a blanket term for health problems that remain after you have recovered from a critical illness. This is due to an array of factors, but it is thought that a mixture of medications, effects of the infection or exacerbation, and isolation may be the culprits. It can take more than a year to recover from post intensive care syndrome. If you have any of the following symptoms, then please reach out to a mental health professional.

Symptoms of Post-Intensive Care Syndrome:
- Problems with critical thinking
- Trouble concentrating
- Trouble problem solving
- Disorganized
- Sleep disturbances
- Nightmares
- Depression
- Anxiety
- Muscle weakness
- Post-traumatic stress disorder (PTSD)

Journal Day 12:

- ❑ Rate both your Mood and Breathing on a scale of 1-10
- ❑ Do you currently have any signs of depression?
- ❑ What about Post-Intensive Care Syndrome?
- ❑ Have you noticed any improvement in your mood since beginning this program?
- ❑ What has been the biggest difference in your mood?

"People who don't know the power of their mind shall only have power without power." - *Ernest Agymemang Yeboah*

◆ ◆ ◆

Day 13 The Power Within

As you have already learned from the dyspnea cycle, anxiety can typically go hand and hand with breathing difficulties. Learning to control your anxiety will not only make your breathing better, but it will make your overall health better as well. While the breathing exercises that you will learn from me will help, when practiced often, it is very likely that you will need to seek guidance from a mental health professional to truly get your anxiety under control. One positive thing that has come out of the pandemic is the increased ability to see mental health professionals via Tele-health from the comfort of your own home! Technology is truly amazing. Anyway, if you do suffer from anxiety and or panic attacks, please seek help from someone trained in doing so.

Not only will anxiety cause your breathing to worsen, but it will also affect other areas of your health. Anxiety can seriously interfere with your quality of life. When your body is stuck in the "fight or flight" mode, then the 'rest and digest' mode is turned off. This is why most people who suffer from breathing problems find themselves also suffering from digestion problems.

Symptoms of Anxiety

- Irritability
- Worrying too much
- Fatigue
- Restlessness
- Muscle tension

- Sleep disturbances (too much or too little)
- Chest tightness
- Shortness of breath
- Racing heart
- tremors
- Headaches
- Indigestion
- Stomach cramps
- Nausea
- Irritable Bowel Disease (IBS)
- Gastroesophageal Reflux Disease

Tips to Deter Anxiety

- Cut out all unnecessary stress
- Learn to say No when you feel overwhelmed
- Learn to ask for help when you need it
- Start each day with seated meditation
- Ask for help from a mental health professional
- Controlled, deep breathing at the beginning of a panic attack

Getting into the habit of daily meditation is one of the best changes you can make. Meditation truly has healing power for the mind, body, and soul. Most people are hesitant to try meditation because it sounds silly or feels strange to them. Please do not let those reasons deter you! With all of these benefits, what is there to lose?

Benefits of Meditation:

- Mood enhancer
- Reduces stress
- Relieves muscle tension
- Promotes healing
- Reduces shortness of breath
- Improves sleep
- Lowers blood pressure
- Lowers heart rate

- Improves memory

Steps

1. Find a quiet and comfortable place to either sit or lie down.
2. Some people find it beneficial to play soft music without words. Meditation music can be found on Amazon in abundance or on a meditation app!
3. Begin by closing your eyes and blocking out any distractions.
4. Find your breath.
5. Notice how your stomach moves in and out like a soft ocean wave.
6. Picture your muscles loosening a little more with each breath
7. Start releasing muscle tension from your head to your feet.
8. Push out any thoughts that try to pop in your head.
9. The only thing that you want to think about is your breath
10. Once your body is completely relaxed, continue to focus on your breathing while you state a positive affirmation, statement, or goal for the day. For Instance, "Today I will remember to breathe." "I will choose to see the positive."
11. When ready, open your eyes
12. Take the time to bring your awareness back to your surroundings...

YouTube is FULL of guided meditation videos. Simply type "Guided Meditation for Beginners" into the YouTube search engine and find a video that you enjoy!

◆ ◆ ◆

Journal Day 13:

- Rate your Mood and Breathing from 1-10
- What symptoms of anxiety do you have?
- How did you enjoy meditation?
- How many days a week can you commit to meditation?

"The first wealth is health." - Ralph Waldo Emerson

Day 14 Rest And Digest

Yesterday I mentioned how your body's nervous system gets itself stuck in the "fight or flight" mode (sympathetic nervous system) due to repeated episodes of shortness of breath. Overtime, this affects your entire body negatively. Staying in this mode for too long, over a long period can lead to poor blood sugar regulation, fatigue, insomnia, weight gain, anxiety, and depression. The reason for this is that if your body's sympathetic nervous system is stimulated, then the parasympathetic nervous system is not. Both modes cannot be on at the same time!

Where the sympathetic nervous system is sometimes called the "fight or flight" mode, the parasympathetic nervous system is called the "rest and digest" mode. The parasympathetic nervous system is responsible for digestion, detoxification, building immunity, regeneration, and healing. Everyone asks me why they are overly tired, bloated, or suffer from indigestion and excess weight. This is the answer! .Think about that for a second...

So, if your body is stuck in its "fight or flight" mode, you're missing out on ALL OF THE GOOD STUFF!!! Your body has natural healing mechanisms, but they must have the time and opportunity to work!!!

The **power is within you** to switch your "fight or flight" mode off. I encourage you to make a conscious effort to slow down and allow yourself time to heal. Break your old, unhealthy patterns of worry and stress. Along with your breathing exercises and meditation, try Tai Chi or Yoga. You do not even have to go to a class. Type "Seated Tai Chi" or "Seated Yoga" into your YouTube search engine and you will find hundreds of videos that you can do from the comfort of your own home! I encourage you to try a seated yoga or tai chi video today! You will not be sorry!

Journal Day 14:

- ❑ Rate your Mood and Breathing on a scale from 1-10
- ❑ Now that you know the function of the parasympathetic nervous system, what problems do you have that could be caused from your body's inability to stay in that mode?
- ❑ What changes can you commit to making to improve your body's natural healing properties?
- ❑ On a personal note, have your needs been being met better than before you started the program?
- ❑ Have you interacted in your Facebook Group? If not, I encourage you to be interactive and make friends. Some of the strongest friendships come from sharing struggles and overcoming them together!

"You are what you eat so don't be fast, cheap, easy, or fake." - Unknown

Day 15 The Nitty Gritty On Food

You now know the importance of slowing your body down so that it has the opportunity to "rest and digest." Now let's talk nutrition!

Believe it or not, nutrition plays a large role in how you breathe. Eating the proper nutrients will help your lungs in several ways! Never underestimate the power a healthy diet can play on your overall health. It will help if you begin to think of food as fuel for your body or possibly, all natural medicine for your body. There is no doubt that you get out what you put in. To begin with, if you happen to be a little overweight, then it would be in your best interest to lose the extra weight. Any extra weight on your neck, chest, or abdomen can cause your breathing to be more difficult. Actually, excess fat decreases respiratory compliance, increases pulmonary resistance, and reduces respiratory muscle strength due to being overworked. That being said, I know it is easier said than done!

Rather than go over ways to lose weight, I want to talk about how to develop healthier eating habits. At the end of the day, that should be your overall goal where nutrition is concerned. It is best to keep a food journal of what you eat. In the journal you should not only write down what you eat, but how the foods make you feel and more importantly, how they affect your breathing. Then think about a couple of tangible weekly goals to work towards and write them down too. Start out by making small changes weekly like swapping one food for another. The key is to eat a well-balanced diet. If you have a smartphone, then download a meal tracker app and it will guide you! You can also speak to a nutritionist if you need more one on one guidance.

If you suffer from breathing issues, then there are some things to consider when you are thinking about changing your diet. Research shows that eating the proper nutrients can help protect your lungs and even reduce lung damage.

For starters, cutting back on your carbohydrate intake will benefit anyone with breathing problems. Foods high in carbohydrates (carbs) produce large amounts of carbon dioxide, which can be toxic if it builds up in your blood. That being said, carbs should not be completely eliminated from your diet because carbs also turn into energy! Try cutting back on the simple carbs like sugary drinks, baked goods, and sweets. Try to add carbs that are also high in fiber like oats or certain beans. Berries of any kind are also perfect carbs to add to your diet, as they are also antioxidants! In fact, adding antioxidants like vitamins A, C, and E have been shown to contribute to the neutralization of those free radicals that destroy lung cells so eat up!

Inflammation is a huge factor in breathing problems. Inflammation is a natural immune response from your body. When your lungs are inflamed, they create more mucus and your airways are narrower. This is why eating foods with natural anti-inflammatory properties is a good dietary move to make. If you happen to have a gluten intolerance, then eating anything containing gluten can cause inflammation throughout your body, including your lungs. Certain preservatives have also been linked to inflammation so eating whole foods is always best! Try eating foods that show the ingredients as having five or less items. Shopping around the outer parts of your local grocery store will keep you in the right sections!

So, we've gone over carbs, antioxidants, and inflammatory foods. Now let us talk a little bit about mucus producing foods. That is right, what you eat and drink can affect the amount of mucus that your body produces! A normal amount of mucus is essential as it protects the mucus membranes in our lungs and prevents foreign bodies from entering our lungs by acting as a trap. We do not want to stop all mucus production, but do want to cut down on mucus in excess and mucus that is too thick. Too much mucus in your body can lead to an infection and difficulty breathing. There are several easy dietary changes that you can make to cut down on the excess and thick mucus. Simply drinking the appropriate amount of water per day will help to thin the mucus that your body produces. You can also cut back on or eliminate mucus producing drinks and foods. Dairy, for example, should be limited for anyone with breathing problems. Dairy products can produce histamine, cause inflammation, and increase mucus production. There are many yummy dairy free products available. Almond milk is delicious and nutritious! You have your work cut out for you, but I have made several lists that may be helpful!

Simple (BAD) Carbohydrates to cut
- Sugar
- Candy
- Pastries
- White bread
- Fruit juice
- Pepsi/coke
- Muffins
- Cookies
- Sugary Cereal

Complex (GOOD) Carbohydrates
- Oats
- Fruits (berries are best)
- Sweet potato
- Peas
- Carrots
- Squash
- Celery
- Broccoli

- Brown rice
- Quinoa
- Nuts/seeds

Antioxidant rich foods (GOOD)
- Blueberries, raspberries, and blackberries
- Turmeric
- Carrots
- Garlic
- Broccoli
- Onions
- Green tea
- Apricot
- Kiwi

Anti-inflammatory foods (GOOD)
- Strawberries & blueberries
- Cherries
- Fish (salmon, mackerel, tuna, and sardines)
- Olive oil
- Nuts (almonds and walnuts)
- Beans
- Lentils

Inflammatory foods (BAD)
- Processed meats (cold cuts)
- Soda
- Refined carbohydrates
- Fried foods

Mucus producing foods (BAD)
- Dairy products
- Deep fried foods
- Corn
- Cookies
- Sugary cereals

Mucus decreasing foods (GOOD)

- Lemons
- Ginger
- Pineapple
- Asparagus
- Celery
- Cauliflower
- Green leafy vegetables

Food Containing Histamine (BAD)
- Dairy products
- Processed foods

*** TIP: *Green Tea contains antioxidants and helps reduce inflammation in the lungs!* ***

Journal Day 15:

- ❑ Rate your Mood and Breathing from 1-10.
- ❑ What food changes do you need to make to correct your eating habits?
- ❑ What did you learn about food that you did not know before?
- ❑ What is one positive nutrition change that you can make this week?

"Failure will never overtake me if my determination to suc-ceed is strong enough." - Og Mandino

Day 16 Commit To Be Fit

Today is all about fitness! The stronger you are, the healthier you are, and the happier you are! Go through these exercises once. If you feel good after one rotation, then go ahead and complete it again! Do up to 3 rounds. You can follow the video on YouTube titles "Breathe Better Seated Exercises with Cardio..." or click on the following link https://youtu.be/Hv4m_NRg5HI

SIDE STRETCH
1. Raise your right hand into the sky while holding on to your chair with your left hand.
2. Inhale through your nose and exhale as you reach your right hand over your head towards the opposite wall until you feel a stretch in your side.
3. Inhale as you come back up and release your arm.
4. Repeat this on your left side.
5. Do this on each side X 3

SHOULDER ROLLS
1. Roll your shoulders in a circular motion backwards 10 times and then change
   directions rolling your shoulders forward 10 X's

SHOULDER SHRUGS
1. Lift your shoulders up and down X 5

GENTLE NECK STRETCH

1. Sitting up straight, slowly tilt your head to the right, bringing your right ear to your right shoulder until you feel a stretch in the left side of your neck.
2. Hold for 5 seconds.
3. Repeat on the other side.
4. Do both sides X 3

SIDE BEND

1. Sit in a comfortable position with your feet flat on the floor
2. Place your hands behind your head, elbows pointing out, even with your shoulders
3. Inhale through your nose, pushing your belly out
4. Exhale slowly as you bend your torso to the right, right elbow facing the floor to the right
5. Inhale as you rise back up to initial position
6. Repeat X 2

LUMBAR ROTATION

1. Cross arms placing opposite hands on the opposite shoulder.
2. Inhale through your nose
3. Gently turn the trunk of your body to your right on an exhale
4. Inhale as you come back to the starting position
5. Gently turn the trunk of your body to your left on an exhale
6. Inhale as you come back to the starting position
7. Repeat on each side X 2

ARM CIRCLES

1. Bring your arms out to a T shape.
2. Move your arms in a circular motion. The circles should be small, like the size
of a dinner plate.
3. Do 10 circles in each direction
4. Repeat X 3, resting in between if needed

ABDUCTIONS
1. Using a 1 lb weight, Bring arms out to a T shape and gently release back down.
2. Do this X 10

BICEP CURLS
1. With or without light weights, drop your arms to your side with palms facing forward
2. Gently curl your arms up by keeping your elbows close to your sides and bending your elbows
3. Do these X 20

ELBOW FLECTION
1. With or without light weights, drop your arms to your sides with palms facing your body, thumbs facing the front
2. Bend your elbows to a 90 degree angle
3. Lower your arms back down to your sides
4. Repeat X 20

SEATED ROWING
1. Sit up straight with your feet firmly on the floor.
2. Reach your arms out in front of you and clasp your hands together with your arms straight.
3. Pull your arms back to one side in a rowing motion with abdominal muscles engaged
4. Repeat on the other side.
5. Do X 10 on each side

SEATED MARCH IN PLACE
1. Sit up tall with a straight back and both feet flat on the floor
2. When ready, left your right leg and left arm
3. Begin marching in place
4. Try to go for 30 seconds to begin with. If this is too easy you can apply an ankle weight or go for longer in 15 second increments

5. Rest for 30 seconds
6. Repeat marching for 30 seconds

SEATED LEG CIRCLES

1. Hold on to the seat of your chair for support.
2. Lift and straighten your right leg
3. Draw a circle with your toes in one direction 5 times
4. Change directions for 5
5. Drop your right leg back down
6. Lift and straighten your left leg
7. Draw a circle with your toes in one direction 5 times
8. Change directions for 5
9. Drop your left leg back down
10. Repeat on each leg X 3

SEATED JUMPING JACKS

1. Begin with knees bent and arms by your sides
2. Extend your legs straight and to the sides with your heals on the floor, while your arms shoot up to a V shape
3. Bring your arms and legs back down
4. Repeat X 10

Journal Day 16:

- ❑ Rate both your Mood and Breathing on a scale of 1-10
- ❑ Can you feel your body getting stronger?
- ❑ How are your breathing exercises going?

"To ensure good health: eat lightly, breathe deeply, live moderately, cultivate cheerfulness, and maintain an interest in life." - William Londen

Day 17 Head Over Meals

To aid in digestion, it is best to spread your meals out. Eat less food more frequently. Break your larger meals into smaller meals. This will decrease bloating by decreasing the size of your stomach following meals. Without your stomach pushing up on your lungs, your lungs and diaphragm will have more room to expand. You may also want to take a gas pill before eating and avoid foods that cause you indigestion.

I am including many yummy recipes in the appendix as well!

Breakfast Ideas:
- Oatmeal with blueberries, strawberries, or raspberries
- Turkey sausage links or patties
- Whole grain toast with nut butter
- Boiled egg
- Egg white omelet with spinach
- Almond milk based smoothie

THINK WHOLE GRAINS, BERRIES, LEAN MEAT

Lunch Ideas:
- Grilled Chicken
- Salad
- Avocado whole grain toast ***My Personal Favorite- try adding "Everything But the Bagel" seasoning!***
- Tuna

AVOID COLD CUTS

Snack Ideas:
- Fresh fruit
- Peppers with hummus - ***My Personal Favorite!***
- Celery and nut butter
- Apples and nut butter
- Nuts
- Hard boiled eggs

AVOID PREPACKAGED SNACKS

Dinner Ideas:
- Salmon - ***My Personal favorite***
- Roasted vegetables
- Gluten free pasta (LIMIT)
- Cauliflower pizza
- Grilled, roasted, or baked chicken
- Grilled, roasted, or bakes turkey
- Sweet potato

AVOID FRIED FOODS

Dessert (My Favorite Meal of the Day) Ideas:
- Fruit with honey, whipped cream, or cool whip
- Dark chocolate
- Frozen bananas dipped in dark chocolate
- Frozen berries dipped in dark chocolate
- Dairy free ice cream
- Frozen fruit bars

Journal Day 17:

- Rate both your Mood and Breathing on a scale of 1-10.
- What will you be having for dinner tonight?

- On a personal note, have you had any moments of clarity during your meditation?
- If so, what have you discovered about yourself?

"There is hope, even when your brain tells you there isn't." - John Green

◆ ◆ ◆

Day 18 Stay Strong, Live Long

While exercise is important, recovery time is equally important. If you do not allow yourself downtime in between strengthening days, then it could actually be worse for your progress. Now, that being said, recovery days are not lazy days! Recovery days are when I recommend gentle stretches, yoga, tai chi, or walking. Here is a weekly example:

- ★ MONDAY - breathing exercises, gentle stretching, strengthening exercises
- ★ TUESDAY - breathing exercises, gentle stretching, yoga, tai chi, or walking
- ★ WEDNESDAY - breathing exercises, gentle stretching, strengthening exercises
- ★ THURSDAY - breathing exercises, gentle stretching, yoga, tai chi, or walking
- ★ FRIDAY - breathing exercises, gentle stretching, strengthening exercises
- ★ SATURDAY - You choose your favorite form of exercise!!!
- ★ SUNDAY - REST

Here you can find today's strengthening exercises by typing in "Breathe Better Seated Exercises with Cardio & Standing..." or click on the following link: **https://youtu.be/Hv4m_NRg5HI**

SIDE STRETCH
1. Raise your right hand into the sky while holding on to your chair with your left hand.
2. Inhale through your nose and exhale as you reach your right hand over your head towards the opposite wall

until you feel a stretch in your side.

3. Inhale as you come back up and release your arm.
4. Repeat this on your left side.
5. Do this on each side X 3

SHOULDER ROLLS

1. Roll your shoulders in a circular motion backwards 10 times and then change

directions rolling your shoulders forward 10 times.

2. Doing shoulder rolls daily will help keep your shoulders loose and making it

easier for your lungs to expand, which will make it easier to breathe.

SHOULDER SHRUGS

1. Lift your shoulders up and down X 5

GENTLE NECK STRETCH

1. Sitting up straight, slowly tilt your head to the right, bringing your right ear to your right shoulder until you feel a stretch in the left side of your neck.
2. Hold for 5 seconds.
3. Repeat on the other side.
4. Do both sides X 3

SIDE BEND

1. Sit in a comfortable position with your feet flat on the floor
2. Place your hands behind your head, elbows pointing out, even with your shoulders
3. Inhale through your nose, pushing your belly out
4. Exhale slowly as you bend your torso to the right, right elbow facing the floor to the right
5. Inhale as you rise back up to initial position

LUMBAR ROTATION

1. Cross arms placing opposite hands on the opposite

shoulder.
2. Inhale through your nose
3. Gently turn the trunk of your body to your right on an exhale
4. Inhale as you come back to the starting position
5. Gently turn the trunk of your body to your left on an exhale
6. Inhale as you come back to the starting position
7. Repeat on each side X 2

ARM CIRCLES
1. Bring your arms out to a T shape.
2. Move your arms in a circular motion. The circles should be small, like the size of a dinner plate.
3. Do 10 in circles in each direction
4. Repeat X 3, resting in between if needed

ABDUCTIONS
1. Using a 1 lb weight, Bring arms out to a T shape and gently release back down.
2. Do this X 10

BICEP CURLS
1. With or without light weights, drop your arms to your side with palms facing forward
2. Gently curl your arms up by keeping your elbows close to your sides and bending your elbows
3. Do these X 20

SEATED MARCH IN PLACE
1. Sit up tall with a straight back and both feet flat on the floor
2. When ready, left your right leg and left arm
3. Begin marching in place
4. Try to go for 30 seconds to begin with. If this is too easy you can apply an ankle weight or go for longer in 15 second increments

5. Rest for 30 seconds
6. Repeat marching for 30 seconds

SEATED JUMPING JACKS
1. Begin with knees bent and arms by your sides
2. Extend your legs straight and to the sides with your heals on the floor, while your arms shoot up to a V shape
3. Bring your arms and legs back down
4. Repeat X 10

If you feel like you can exercise while standing, follow these exercises. If you are not quite there yet, no worries, just go back to do day 16 and repeat those exercises instead! Stay seated for however long it takes you to build up enough strength to try the standing exercises. Everyone recovers at a different pace so do not be discouraged! If the following sequence of exercises is easy, add ankle weights.

HEEL RAISES
1. Stand up and hold on to the back of your chair for support
2. Lift both heels off the ground
3. Bring your heels back down
4. Repeat X 20

KICK BACKS
1. Hold on to the back of your chair for support
2. Keeping your left foot on the ground, kick your straightened right leg behind you
3. Repeat X 20
4. Keeping your right foot on the ground, kick your straightened left leg behind you
5. Repeat X 20

SIDE KICKS
1. Hold on to the back of your chair for support
2. Keeping you left foot on the ground, kick your straightened right leg out to your right side

3. Repeat X 20
4. Keeping your right foot on the ground, kick your straightened left leg out to your left side
5. Repeat X 20

SIT TO STAND

1. Sit in your chair with your feet flat on the ground
2. Reach your arms out in front of you
3. Stand up
4. Sit back down
5. Repeat x 20

SQUATS (ONLY IF SIT TO STANDS ARE MASTERED)

1. Stand in front of your chair with your feet hip width apart
2. Reach your arms out in front of you
3. Bend your knees, sit your hips back as if sitting down, but do not touch the chair
4. Straighten up to a standing position
5. Repeat X 10

BENT LEG KICK BACK

1. Hold on to the back of your chair for support
2. Keeping your left foot on the ground, bend your right leg to a 90 degree angle
3. Keeping your leg bent, kick back
4. Repeat X 20
5. Place your right foot on the ground
6. Keeping your right foot on the ground, bend your left leg to a 90 degree angle
7. Keeping your leg bent, kick back
8. Repeat X 20

WALL PUSH UPS

1. Stand facing the wall at arms-length away
2. Place your hands on the wall, shoulder width apart
3. Bend your elbows as you lean your face towards the wall

4. Slowly push back to your starting position
5. Repeat X 10

★ Repeat this entire series up to 2 more times as tolerated.

Journal Day 18:

❑ Rate your Mood and Breathing on a scale of 1-10
❑ What has been your favorite part of the program so far?
❑ What changes have you noticed in your breathing?

"Every single thing you go through is designed to GROW you. Every experience made you who you are today." - Unknown

◆ ◆ ◆

Day 19 Protection From Infection

When your lungs have had significant infection like COVID-19, there is more than likely lung damage. The same is true for COPD and other lung diseases. When you have had lung damage, it is much easier for you to catch an upper respiratory infection. The same infection that causes your friend to have an intermittent cough can cause a severe infection in you that may even require hospitalization. Each time that you have a serious lung infection or exacerbation, your lungs will get a little worse. It is so important that you make changes to prevent infections!

Tips to Prevent Infection
- Find your triggers and avoid them!
- Wash your hands often!
- Wear your mask in public during cold and flu season
- Stay current on ALL vaccines
- Don't touch your face
- Brush your teeth at least twice a day
- Eat a nutritious healthy diet
- Learn to recognize the early warning signs of an infection

Early Warning Signs- When to Call your MD
- Increased cough frequency
- Changes in mucus production
- Changes in mucus color (normal is clear to white)
- Increased shortness of breath (journaling will come in handy

here)
- More frequent use of your rescue inhaler
- Lack of appetite
- Increased fatigue
- Swelling in the ankles, legs, around eyes
- Lowering oxygen levels
- Fever

When to Call 911
- Chest pain
- Confusion
- Vision problems
- Unable to speak due to sudden shortness of breath
- Blue lips and nail beds
- Coughing up blood

Do not exercise if you have symptoms of a respiratory infection. You should conserve your energy. You do however want to continue your deep breathing exercises.

Journal Day 19:

- Rate Mood and Breathing on a scale of 1-10
- Are there any changes that you can make to prevent an infection?
- How is your breathing coming along?
- What improvements have you noticed in your breathing?
- What about your endurance?

"Healing doesn't mean the damage never existed. It means the damage no longer controls our lives." - Unknown

◆ ◆ ◆

Day 20 Put One Foot In Front Of The Other

It is time to start putting one foot in front of the other. The absolute, very best form of exercise is walking! Walking engages your entire body all at once. According to the National Heart Lung and Blood Institute, regular, brisk 30-minute walks increase lung capacity. This will obviously cause you to breathe better!

Walking is perfect for almost everyone. It benefits your entire body. It's easy on your joints, strengthens your joints, improves your mood, improves circulation, essential for heart health, lowers blood pressure, helps regulate blood sugar levels, aids in digestion, increases your metabolism, burns calories, strengthens bones, improves shortness of air, increases endurance, reduces belly fat, reduces muscle tension, reduces stress, and promotes a good night's sleep! With all of these benefits, how can you resist?

If walking is difficult for you now, continue your seated exercises and add seated marching for the length of time that you would be walking. As you build strength in your legs, walking will become easier. I have developed a simple and effective walking plan that you can use to build strength and endurance. The key is to start wherever you can physically and then build up on a weekly basis. You should always be able to carry on a conversation as you walk. If you are unable to speak due to breathing difficulties, then stop and rest.

Begin by walking for 2-5 minutes as tolerated. If you are unable to walk, then do seated marching in place or standing marching in place for 2-5 minutes as tolerated. Walk at a minimum of 3 days per week.

Every week add 1 minute to your walking. Keep adding 1 minute a week until you are up to 20-45 minutes as tolerated. With breathing problems, this may not be possible every day. It is important that you let yourself take a break or skip the walking altogether if you do not feel up to walking due to your shortness of air. Following a walking plan will improve your quality of life and exercise capacity so please keep it up! Remember that **the power is within you** to change!

Journal Day 20:

- ❏ Rate your Mood and Breathing from 1-10.
- ❏ How do you feel when you walk?
- ❏ Do you struggle with walking?
- ❏ Do you need to build up endurance?

"Every new beginning comes from some other beginning's end."
- Seneca

Day 21 On To New Beginnings

Congratulations, you have trudged forward and reached the end of this journey. It may be the end of our journey together, but it is the beginning of yours. It is imperative that you continue on your journey of healing from here on out. You have the knowledge and the strength needed to manage your symptoms and build on the foundation that we have built over the last 21 days.

My hope is that you have grown not only to love yourself again, but also to see yourself as bigger than your challenges or limitations. I encourage you to stay strong, persevere, and continue on your path to self-discovery. Live each day with a purpose as you see it.

Just remember, **the power is in you** and **it always has been.**

Journal Day 21
- ❏ Rate your Mood and Breathing on a scale of 1-10.
- ❏ What is the most fulfilling thing you've learned over the last 21 days?
- ❏ How has your breathing changed over the last 21 days?
- ❏ Write down a schedule of meditation, strengthening, and walking that you know you can stick to.

Appendix

Inhaler to Nebulizer Conversion List for Cost Savings

Prescribed:	Equivalent nebulizer:
1. ProAir HFA	1. Albuterol
2. Arcapta Neohaler	2. Brovana (arformoterol)
Serevent, Foradil	15 mcg nebulizer
3. Atrovent	3. Atrovent (Ipratropium
Spiriva	Bromide) 0.5mg
Tudorza	
Incruse Ellipta	

4. Fluticasone Furoate   4. Pulmicort (Budesonide)
    Beclomethasone   0.5mg
    Triamcinolone
    Budesonide
    Mometasone

5. Combivent Respimat   5. DuoNeb (albuterol/
   (albuterol/ipratropium)   ipratropium)

6. Advair   6. Pulmicort 0.5mg +
   Symbicort   Brovana 15mcg
   Dulera
   Breo Ellipta

7. Anoro Ellipta   7. Atrovent 0.5mg +
   Ultibro Neohaler   Brovana 15mcg
   Stilolto Respimat

8. Trelegy   8. Brovana + Atrovent + Pulmicort 9.
Daliresp   9. Pulmicort

*** PLEASE NOTE THAT THESE CONVERSIONS ARE FOR COST SAVING MEASURES ONLY. THE DOSAGES AND DIRECTIONS WILL VARY. SOME OF THE CONVERSIONS ARE NOT EXACT AND YOU MAY BENEFIT MORE FROM THE INHALER FORM.***

BORG SCALE 1-10

0 - REST
1 - REALLY EASY
2 - EASY
3 - MODERATE
4 - SORT OF HARD
5 - HARD
6 - HARD
7 - REALLY HARD
8 - REALLY HARD
9 - REALLY, REALLY, HARD
10 - MAXIMAL EXERTION

◆ ◆ ◆

LUNG HEALTHY BREAKFAST SMOOTHIE RECIPES

◆ ◆ ◆

Immunity Tart

INGREDIENTS

- 3 oranges, juiced
- 1/3 c freshly squeezed lemon juice
- 1 tbsp. raw agave
- 1 -inch piece of ginger root, peeled and chopped
- 1/8 tsp. cayenne pepper

- 1/2 c chopped pineapple, frozen overnight
- 1 tbsp. coconut oil
- 5 mint leaves

INSTRUCTIONS

1. Add everything to a blender and blend untilsmooth. If you want it a little thicker, you can add some ice cubes and blend until you have reached your desired consistency.
2. If you would prefer it creamier, add almond milk.
3. Serve immediately and enjoy.

Awesome In A Cup

INGREDIENTS

- 2 cups freshly squeezed orange juice, or equal quantity peeled and pitted oranges
- 1 unpeeled, pitted apple
- 1 ripe banana
- ½ cup blueberries
- 1 teaspoon turmeric
- A pinch of pepper
- 1 teaspoon cinnamon
- 3 tablespoons of almond butter
- 3 brazil nuts
- 2 teaspoons fresh grated ginger
- 3 teaspoons chia seeds

INSTRUCTIONS

1. Blend all ingredients until smooth.

2. Drink!

Strawberry & Banana Explosion

Ingredients
- 1 1/2 cup strawberries
- 1 large banana
- 2 cups pineapple juice
- 3 tablespoons oats
- 2 brazil nuts or 4 almonds
- 1/2 teaspoon cardamom or cinnamon
- 1 teaspoon dried stinging nettle
- 1 teaspoon maca powder

INSTRUCTIONS
1. Transfer all of the ingredients to the bowl of your blender and blend until smooth.
2. Can mix with almond milk if you prefer it to be creamier.
3. Drink!

Green Machine

INGREDIENTS

- 3/4 cup ice
- 1 cup lightly packed spinach leaves
- 2/3 cup plain yogurt (low-fat or whole milk, see NOTE)
- 1/2 cup sliced almonds
- 1 very ripe medium pear (any variety), peeled, cored and cut into chunks
- 3 pitted dates, coarsely chopped
- 1 1/2 teaspoons chopped fresh ginger
- Honey, to taste (optional)

INSTRUCTION

1. Place the ice into a blender and process to crush it.

2. Add the spinach, yogurt, almonds, pear, dates, ginger, and blend until smooth and frothy, with a little texture remaining from the almonds and dates.

3. Taste and then blend in a little honey to taste, if desired.

Lung Healthy Lunch Recipes

Anti-Inflammatory Pumpkin Soup

INGREDIENTS
- 2 tablespoons red curry paste
- 4 cups chicken or vegetable broth about 32 ounces
- 2 15 ounce cans pumpkin puree
- 1 3/4 cup coconut milk or a 13.5 ounce can, reserving 1 tablespoon
- 1 large red chili pepper sliced
- cilantro for garnish if desired

INSTRUCTIONS

1. In a large saucepan over medium heat, cook the curry paste for about one minute or until paste becomes fragrant. Add the broth and the pumpkin and stir.
2. Cook for about 3 minutes or until soup starts to bubble. Add the coconut milk and cook until hot, about 3 minutes.
3. Ladle into bowls and garnish with a drizzle of the reserved coconut milk and sliced red chili's. Garnish with cilantro leaves if desired.

Red, White, And Blue Antioxidant Salad

INGREDIENTS

- 1 pint strawberries, hulled and quartered
- 1 pint blueberries
- ½ cup white sugar (or sugar substitute)
- 2 tablespoons lemon juice
- 4 bananas

INSTRUCTIONS

1. Mix the strawberries and blueberries together in a bowl,
2. Sprinkle with sugar and lemon juice
3. Toss lightly
4. Refrigerate until cold, at least 30 minutes
5. Cut the bananas into 3/4-inch thick slices
6. Toss with the berries.

Avocado Salad

INGREDIENTS

- 1 teaspoon Dijon mustard
- ¼ cup extra-virgin olive oil
- ½ cup balsamic vinegar
- 1 pinch ground black pepper

- 1 avocado - peeled, pitted and sliced
- 2 small tomatoes, each cut into 8 wedges

INSTRUCTIONS

1. In a small bowl, whisk together the mustard, olive oil, balsamic vinegar and pepper.
2. Arrange the slices of avocado and tomato alternately like the spokes of a wheel on one big serving plate, or individual plates.
3. Drizzle lightly with the dressing, and serve immediately.

Lung Healthy Dinner Recipes

Rosemary Crusted Salmon

INGREDIENTS

- 2 teaspoons Dijon mustard
- 1 clove garlic, minced
- ¼ teaspoon lemon zest
- 1 teaspoon lemon juice
- 1 teaspoon chopped fresh rosemary
- ½ teaspoon honey
- ½ teaspoon kosher salt
- ¼ teaspoon crushed red pepper
- 3 tablespoons panko breadcrumbs
- 3 tablespoons finely chopped walnuts
- 1 teaspoon extra-virgin olive oil
- 1 (1 pound) skinless salmon fillet, fresh or frozen
- Olive oil cooking spray
- Chopped fresh parsley and lemon wedges for garnish

INSTRUCTIONS

1. Preheat oven to 425 degrees F. Line a large rimmed baking sheet with parchment paper
2. Combine mustard, garlic, lemon zest, lemon juice, rosemary, honey, salt and crushed red pepper in a small bowl. Combine panko, walnuts, and oil in another small bowl.

3. Place salmon on the prepared baking sheet. Spread the mustard mixture over the fish and sprinkle with the panko mixture, pressing to adhere. Lightly coat with cooking spray.

4. Bake until the fish flakes easily with a fork, about 8 to 12 minutes, depending on thickness.

5. Sprinkle with parsley and serve with lemon wedges, if desired.

Shrimp And Vegetables

INGREDIENTS

- 3 TBSP butter or coconut oil
- 1 onion sliced
- 1 cup coconut milk
- 1-3 tsp curry powder
- 1 lb shrimp tails removed
- 1 bag frozen cauliflower or other frozen veggi

Instructions

1. Melt butter or oil in a skillet and add sliced onion.
2. Sauté onion until it is slightly soft
3. Meanwhile, steam vegetables.
4. When onion is softened, add coconut milk, curry seasoning, and other spices if desired.
5. Cook for a couple minutes to incorporate flavors.
6. Add thawed shrimp and cook approximately 5 minutes or until shrimp are cooked
7. Serve with steamed veggies of choice topped with butter and salad with homemade dressing.

Lung Healthy Dessert Recipes

Homemade Dark Chocolate

INGREDIENTS

- ½ cup coconut oil
- ½ cup cocoa powder
- 3 tablespoons honey
- ½ teaspoon vanilla extract

INSTRUCTIONS

1. Gently melt coconut oil in a saucepan over medium-low heat.
2. Stir cocoa powder, honey, and vanilla extract into melted oil until well blended.
3. Pour mixture into a candy mold or pliable tray.
4. Refrigerate until chilled, about 1 hour.

Healthy Apple Pie With A Twist

Ingredients

- CRUST

- oil for greasing the pan (I use a non-stick spray, but olive, coconut, or grapeseed oil is also fine)
- 1 1/4 cup toasted walnuts
- 3/4 cup old fashioned rolled oats
- 1/4 teaspoon salt
- 3/4 cup + 2 tablespoons whole wheat pastry flour or spelt flour
- 3 tablespoons coconut oil
- 1/4 cup maple syrup
- 1 teaspoon vanilla extract
- FILLING
- 1 1/2 cup + 2 teaspoons apple juice
- 1 1/2 teaspoon agar powder
- 1 1/2 teaspoon arrowroot powder
- 4 medium granny smith apples or pears
- 1 lemon
- 1 teaspoon cinnamon
- 1/2 teaspoon freshly ground nutmeg or 1/4 teaspoon nutmeg powder
- 1 tablespoon maple syrup or brown sugar
- 1/2 teaspoon vanilla extract
- 1 orange

Instructions

1. Preheat oven to 350°, and grease a tart pan.
2. In a food processor blend the oats, walnuts, salt, and flour until it resembles a coarse meal.
3. Then pour in maple syrup, coconut oil, and vanilla, and blend again. You should have a sticky damp dough. Be careful not to over blend.
4. Press and shape the walnut dough into the tart pan. Make sure the walls are thick enough and packed tightly.

5. Poke holes into the bottom with a fork and bake for 15 minutes at 350°.

FILLING

1. Peel, core, and thinly slice the apples. Squeeze the juice of a lemon over the apple slices to prevent browning.
2. Pour 1 cup of apple juice and agar powder into a pan, whisk well. Bring it to a simmer and continue to cook for 5 minutes, covered.
3. In a small bowl mix the arrowroot powder and the remaining 2 teaspoons of apple juice. Stir well to eliminate any chunks. Pour it into the cooking agar mixture, and whisk for a few minutes until it begins to thicken. It will not thicken too much, and will still be liquidy. Then remove it from the heat.
4. To the apple slices, add nutmeg, cinnamon, maple syrup, and vanilla. Use your hands to toss them.
5. Configure the apples into the center of the baked piecrust, and then pour the agar mixture evenly over the apples.
6. To avoid burnt edges, cover the edges in aluminum foil.
7. Bake for 40-45 minutes, until the apples are tender.
8. Let it cool a bit before serving warm or room temperature. Garnish with orange zest before serving.

Made in United States
Troutdale, OR
12/31/2024

27465537R00056